HOW TO
EAT

THICH NHAT HANH

PARALLAX
PRESS

Berkeley, California

Parallax Press
P.O. Box 7355
Berkeley, California 94710
www.parallax.org

Parallax Press is the publishing division of
Unified Buddhist Church, Inc.
© 2014 by Unified Buddhist Church
All rights reserved
Printed in The United States of America

Cover and text design by Debbie Berne
Illustrations by Jason DeAntonis

ISBN: 978-1-937006-72-3

Library of Congress Cataloging-in-Publication Data
Nhat Hanh, Thich, author.
  How to eat / Thich Nhat Hanh ; illustrated by Jason
DeAntonis.
    pages cm
  ISBN 978-1-937006-72-3 (paperback)
1. Meditation—Buddhism. 2. Dinners and dining—
Religious aspects—Buddhism. I. Title.
  BQ9800.T5392N45448 2014
  294.3'444—dc23
                                    2014015222

1 2 3 4 5 / 18 17 16 15 14

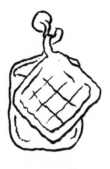

CONTENTS

NOTES ON EATING

MINDFUL EATING

To cultivate mindfulness, we can do the same things we always do—walking, sitting, working, eating, and so on—with mindful awareness of what we are doing. When we're eating, we know that we are eating. When we open a door, we know that we're opening a door. Our mind is with our actions.

When you put a piece of fruit into your mouth, all you need is a little bit of mindfulness to be aware: "I am putting a piece of apple in my mouth." Your mind doesn't need to be somewhere else. If you're thinking of work while you chew, that's not eating mindfully. When you pay attention to the apple, that is mindfulness. Then you can look more deeply and in just a very short time you will see the apple seed, the beautiful orchard and the sky, the farmer, the picker, and so on. A lot of work is in that apple!

NOTHING COMES
FROM NOTHING

With just a little bit of mindfulness, you can
truly see where your bread comes from. It has
not come from nothing. Bread comes from
the wheat fields, from hard work, and from the
baker, the supplier, and the seller. But the bread
is more than that. The wheat field needs clouds
and sunshine. So in this slice of bread there is
sunshine, there is cloud, there is the labor of the
farmer, the joy of having flour, and the skill of
the baker and then—miraculously!—there is the
bread. The whole cosmos has come together
so that this piece of bread can be in your hand.
You don't need to do a lot of hard work to get
this insight. You only need to stop letting your
mind carry you away with worrying, thinking,
and planning.

YOUR BODY BELONGS
TO THE EARTH

In modern life, people tend to think their bodies belong to them, that they can do anything they want to themselves. But your body is not only yours. Your body belongs to your ancestors, your parents, and future generations. It also belongs to society and to all the other living beings. The trees, the clouds, the soil, and every living thing brought about the presence of your body. We can eat with care, knowing we are caretakers of our bodies, rather than their owners.

EATING WITHOUT THINKING

When we eat we usually think. We can enjoy our eating a lot more if we practice not thinking when we eat. We can just be aware of the food. Sometimes we eat and we're not aware that we're eating. Our mind isn't there. When our mind isn't present, we look but we don't see, we listen but we don't hear, we eat but we don't know the flavor of the food. This is a state of forgetfulness, the lack of mindfulness. To be truly present we have to stop our thinking. This is the secret of success.

WAITING WITHOUT WAITING

When we serve ourselves food and then bring it to the table, we don't need to feel we're waiting for other people to serve themselves and be seated. All we have to do is breathe and enjoy sitting. We haven't eaten our meal yet, but we can already feel joy and gratitude. It's an opportunity for us to be peaceful.

Standing in line at a grocery store or a restaurant, or waiting for the time to eat, we don't need to waste our time. We don't need to "wait" for one second. Instead, we can enjoy breathing in and out for our nourishment and healing. We can use that time to notice that we will soon be able to have food, and we can be happy and grateful during that time. Instead of waiting, we can generate joy.

SLOWING DOWN

When we can slow down and really enjoy our food, our life takes on a much deeper quality. I love to sit and eat quietly and enjoy each bite, aware of the presence of my community, aware of all the hard and loving work that has gone into my food. When I eat in this way, not only am I physically nourished, I am also spiritually nourished. The way I eat influences everything else that I do during the day.

Eating is as important a time for meditation as sitting or walking mediation time. It's a chance to receive the many gifts of the Earth that I would not otherwise benefit from if my mind were elsewhere. Here is a verse I like to recite when I eat:

In the dimension of space and time,
We chew as rhythmically as we breathe.
Maintaining the lives of all our ancestors,
Opening an upward path for descendants.

We can use the time of eating to nourish the best things our relatives have passed onto us and to transmit what is most precious to future generations.

PAYING ATTENTION
TO JUST TWO THINGS

While we eat, we can try to pay attention to just two things: the food that we're eating and our friends who are sitting around us and eating with us. This is called mindfulness of food and mindfulness of community. Eating mindfully, we become aware of all the work and energy that has gone into bringing the food to us. If we are eating with others, we can notice how wonderful it is that during this sometimes hectic life we can find the time to sit together in a relaxed way like this to enjoy a meal. When you can breathe, sit, and eat together with your family or friends in mindfulness, this is called true community-building.

EACH SPOONFUL CONTAINS THE UNIVERSE

Pay attention to each spoonful of food. As you bring it up to your mouth, use your mindfulness to be aware that this food is the gift of the whole universe. The Earth and the sky have collaborated to bring this spoonful of food to you. While breathing in and out, you only need a second or two to recognize this. We eat in such a way that every morsel of food, every moment of eating has mindfulness in it. It takes only a few seconds to see that the food we're holding in our spoon is the gift of the whole cosmos. While we chew, we maintain that awareness. When we chew, we know that the whole universe is there in that bite of food.

BREATHING COMES FIRST

The first thing to do when you sit down with your bowl of food is to stop the thinking and be aware of your breathing. Breathe in such a way that you are nourished. You are nourished by your breathing and you nourish other people with your practice of breathing. We nourish one another.

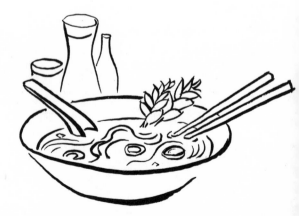

TURNING OFF THE TV

Sometimes people eat while watching TV. But even if you turn off the TV, the TV in your mind continues to run. So you have to also stop the TV in your head. If there is thinking still going on in your mind, you'll be dispersed. To be truly present you need to not just turn off the television or radio in your house, you need to turn off the conversation and images in your head.

HOW MUCH IS ENOUGH

We don't need to eat a lot to feel nourished.
When we are fully there and alive for every
morsel of food, we eat in a way that each bite
fills us with peace and happiness. If we are full
of this joy, we may find that we naturally feel
satisfied with less food.

PREPARING A MEAL

When you prepare a meal with artful awareness, it's delicious and healthy. You have put
your mindfulness, love, and care into the meal,
then people will be eating your love. People
can fully enjoy the meal with body and mind,
just like you enjoy a beautiful work of art.
Eating is not only nourishing for the body, but
also for the mind.

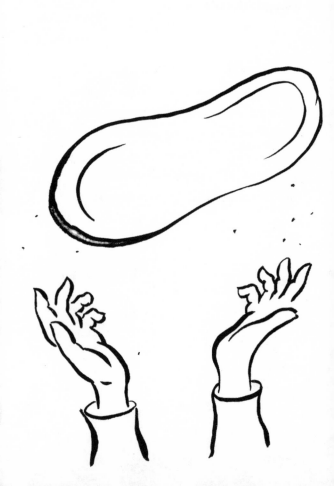

THE KITCHEN

The kitchen can be a meditative practice space if we practice mindful awareness while we are cooking and cleaning there. We can set an intention to execute our tasks in a relaxed and serene way, following our breathing and keeping our concentration on what we are doing. If we are working with others, we may only need to exchange a few words about the work at hand.

A KITCHEN ALTAR

In your own kitchen, you might want to create a kitchen altar to remind yourself to practice mindfulness while cooking. It can be just a small shelf with enough room for an incense holder and perhaps a small flower vase, a beautiful stone, a small picture of an ancestor or spiritual teacher, or a statue—whatever is most meaningful to you. When you come into the kitchen, you can begin your work by offering incense and practicing mindful breathing, making the kitchen into a meditation hall.

COOKING WITHOUT RUSHING

While cooking, allow enough time so you don't feel rushed. If we are aware that our bodies and those of our loved ones depend on the food we're preparing, this awareness will guide us to cook healthy food infused with our love and mindful attention.

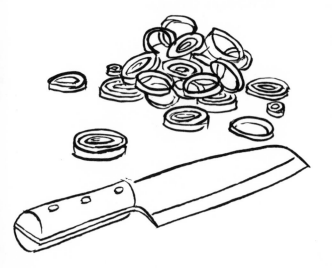

PRACTICING PEACE WHILE CHOPPING VEGETABLES

Peace can be practiced while chopping vegetables, cooking, washing dishes, watering the vegetable garden, and also while driving or working. Practice releasing the tension in body and mind and being completely with your task. The time when you work in the kitchen is also the time for meditation.

SETTING THE TABLE

Eating a meal in mindfulness is an important practice. We turn off the TV, put down our newspaper, and work together for five or ten minutes, setting the table and finishing whatever needs to be done. During these few minutes, we can be very happy. When the food is on the table and eveyone is seated, we practice breathing. "Breathing in, I calm my body. Breathing out, I smile," we repeat three times. We can recover ourselves completely after three breaths like this.

COOKING WITH JOY

Cooking can bring us a lot of joy. When I put the water into the basin for washing the vegetables, I look deeply at the water to see its wonderful nature. I see that the water comes from high in the mountains or from deep within the Earth right into our kitchen. I know that there are places where people have to walk several miles just to carry back a pail of water on their shoulders. Here, water is available whenever I turn on the tap. Aware of the preciousness of clean water, I value the water that is available to me. I also value the electricity that I use to turn on a light or to boil water. I only need to be aware that there is water and electricity easily accessible to me, and I can be happy straightaway. When I am peeling vegetables or cooking them, I can do it in mindfulness and with love. I see cooking as a way to offer nourishment and care to my family and friends. I will easily find joy and peace in the work. Looking deeply at a tomato, a bunch of grapes, or a piece of tofu, I can see the wonderful nature of these things, how they were nurtured by the soil, the sun, the rain, and the seed. Try to organize your life so that you have enough time and energy to cook in a leisurely and peaceful way. The energy of love and harmony in the kitchen will penetrate into the food that you're cooking to offer to your loved ones and yourself.

A GRAIN OF RICE CONTAINS THE UNIVERSE

When we look at a grain of rice, one second of mindfulness and concentration allows us to see that this grain contains the whole world—the rain, the cloud, the Earth, time, space, farmers, everything. Mindfulness and concentration bring insight, and suddenly we can see so much in a grain of rice. It's very quick! Wherever there is mindfulness and concentration, there is insight. When you put that grain of rice into your mouth, you are putting the whole universe in your mouth. This is possible when you stop your thinking. When you chew that grain of rice, just chew, so no thinking will cut you off from this wonderful reality.

COMMUNION

In some traditions, monastics want to take their minds off food and focus on the virtues of a spiritual life. In my tradition, we do the opposite. We just focus on the food. We see the food as the cosmos. In the Catholic tradition, in the Eucharist you see the piece of bread as the body of Jesus. In the Buddhist tradition, we see the piece of bread as the body of the cosmos. Everything is there. When you chew it mindfully, without thinking, you can see very well all that the piece of bread contains. That is why when you take a bite of the bread and chew mindfully, you are truly in communion with all of life.

TAKE YOUR TIME

It's good to take time to eat, because the time
for a meal can be a very happy time. Take time
to enjoy your breakfast, lunch, and dinner.
Enjoy your meal. Stop the thinking and be
there fully, body and mind.

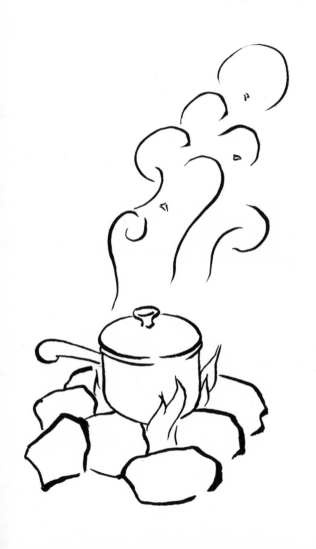

AN AMBASSADOR
OF THE COSMOS

When you pick up an ear of corn, take one second to look at it. You can see the Earth, the sunshine, and the rain in the corn. Everything has come together to produce that corn you are holding. So the corn is an ambassador coming to nourish you. It only takes one or two seconds to get that insight. When you put the corn into your mouth, chew it mindfully and greet the universe.

CHEW YOUR FOOD,
NOT YOUR WORRIES

Sometimes we eat, but we aren't thinking of our food. We're thinking of the past or the future or mulling over some worry or anxiety again and again. So stop thinking about your business, about the office, or about anything that isn't happening right now. Don't chew your worries, your fear, or your anger. If you chew your planning and your anxiety, it's difficult to feel grateful for each piece of food. Just chew your food.

NOURISHED BY THE PRACTICE

Try to be present with your food and with the people sitting around the table with you. Don't close your eyes or look down while you chew. You can open your eyes and if you are with people, notice them alive and well. When we chew with awareness, we're not just nourished by the food, we're nourished by our practice of mindfulness, peace, and happiness. While we chew, we breathe and we enjoy our breathing and our ability to eat and receive nourishment from our food.

FOOD AS MEDICINE

In the original Five Contemplations as they were recited during the Buddha's time, food was considered to be medicine. But I think that when the Buddha received good food, he also enjoyed it. I don't think he thought of it as just taking medicine. We know the food nourishes our bodies. But we can also appreciate and savor our food.

HEALING

When we eat mindfully, we consume exactly what we need in order to keep our bodies, our minds, and the Earth healthy. When we practice like this, we reduce suffering for ourselves and for others. We begin to heal ourselves and can help heal the world. As a spiritual family and as the human family, we can all help make our lives more sustainable by following this practice.

TURNING OFF THE RADIO

In order to eat with joy, we have to turn off
"Radio NST": Non-Stop Thinking. Even if our
bodies are sitting still while we eat, usually
our minds are racing. In order to truly be present for our meal, we have to stop the constant
internal dialogue. To eat without thinking is
to eat in freedom. We are free because we're
not thinking about the past, the future, and our
projects. We are free to be sitting, whether
alone or with loved ones, and enjoying
our meal.

OUR ANCESTORS
ARE IN THE SOIL

That nut, fruit, vegetable, or grain that you eat
has pulled up nutrition from the soil in order
to grow. In the soil are many people who
have died, have been transformed, and have
become part of the soil. Maybe in this mouthful
of rice are also the bones of many hundreds
of generations as well as many dead leaves,
worms, and animals' bones. Maybe in a previ-
ous life you had been there and died there,
and your own bones have disintegrated in that
land. During the time of eating, your practice
is to look deeply into that grain of rice and
enjoy all that has gone into its creation. There
are so many things to enjoy and to discover in
each bite.

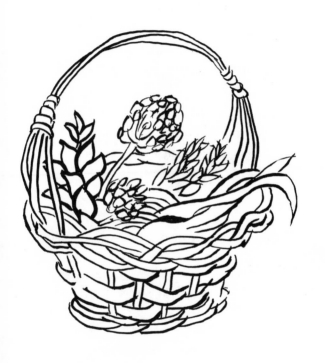

EATING MINDFULLY
IS A PRACTICE

When we eat our meal, we should show up
for that meal 100 percent. Eating mindfully is a
practice. If we choose to drink a cup of tea in
mindfulness, the pleasure of drinking tea will
more than double because we are truly there
and the tea is also truly there. Life is real; it's
not a dream when mindfulness is there.

EATING IN SILENCE

Sometimes, it can be helpful to have a silent meal to help us practice mindful eating. That way, we can focus our attention on our breath, the food, and the company around us in order to become fully present in the here and now.

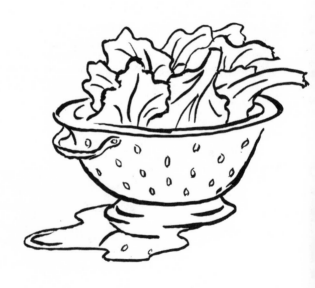

EATING A STRING BEAN

Hold up a string bean and take a moment
to see that it is a string bean with the whole
world in it. There are clouds, sunshine,
the whole Earth, and the hard work of the
gardener. When we can see like that, we
have wisdom. When we have wisdom, it
means that we have mindfulness and concentration. Don't chew your worries, your
suffering, or your projects. That's not good
for your heath. Just chew the string bean.

NOURISHED BY THE PRESENT MOMENT

In our daily activities, we often rush from one thing to another. In between tasks we spend our time planning how we'll accomplish future tasks. In all that hurrying and strategizing, we become isolated from the present moment. Eating is a chance to return to the present moment and stop the rushing and the planning.

HOW THE BUDDHA ATE

Eating meditation is a practice that dates back very far. During his lifetime, the Buddha ate with his community of monks and nuns. Each day they ate together in silence, nourished by the food and by the presence of their brothers and sisters in the practice. I don't think they were worrying about their schedule or about the past or the future. I think they just enjoyed being together and eating well. We can eat like that too.

THE VALUE OF A MEAL

We should reflect deeply on what we buy and what we eat. What we buy and eat can contribute to climate change or it can help stop it. Eating is a chance to nourish our bodies and know that we are not destroying the Earth by doing so.

The value of a meal is not just determined by the amount of money we've spent on the ingredients or on a meal at a restaurant. There is so much hard work that goes into growing, harvesting, distributing, and cooking even a dish of rice. A good meal doesn't have to mean it contains expensive ingredients. The best food is often very simple. There are things the grocery store can't provide us with. No matter how much money you have, you can't buy it.

It's only with mindfulness, concentration, and insight that you can get a truly rich meal.

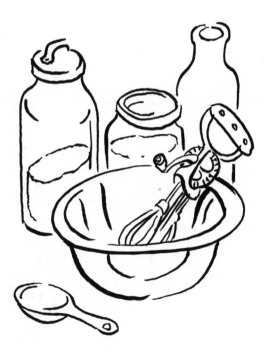

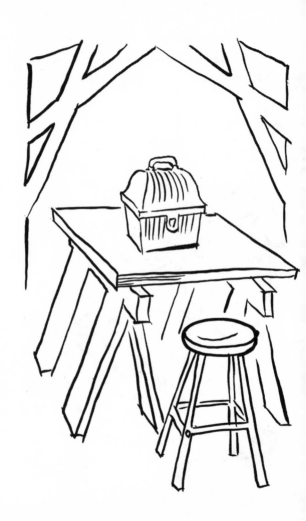

SITTING WHILE YOU EAT

Sometimes we are rushing so much in our day that we eat only as we're running from one place to another. We eat in our car or as we walk. Please sit when you eat. When you sit, that is a reminder to stop. You have nothing to do, nowhere to go.

ONE MINDFUL BREATH

It takes only one moment to take a mindful in-breath and out-breath before you eat.
Bring the mind back to the body. Your body is
always available for you. You can bring your
attention out of your head and into your body.
Before you focus on the food, focus on being
present with your body: "Breathing in, I am
aware that my body is still there. Breathing out,
I smile to my body." This body has been given
to us by our parents and those before them.
When this body was just born, it was very light.
As we grow, we tend to get weighed down by
worries and lose our freshness and beauty.
Mindful eating helps us regain this freshness,
nourishing our spirits as well as our bodies.
Eating with appreciation of our own bodies, we
eat with more relaxation and joy.

THE RIGHT AMOUNT

When we take a moment to sit and breathe before we eat, we can get in touch with the real hunger in our body. We can discover if we're eating because we're hungry or if we're eating because it's the time to eat and the food is there. If we're paying attention and taking our time, we also know how much to eat. Mindfulness is recognizing what is there in the present moment. What is there is the fact that you are still alive and your health is still there. The food in front of you is available to help nourish your body and keep you healthy.

A SILENT MEAL

Happiness is possible during the meal, and silence helps enormously. You may want to pick one meal a week to eat in silence. A silent meal helps you come back to yourself and arrive in the present moment. A truly silent meal includes turning off the noise in your head as well as finding a quiet place to enjoy your meal. You may like to choose to eat the same meal every week silently. This can be a meal you eat by yourself or, if you have family or friends who want to join you for this meal, that is wonderful. Silence helps you return to your mindful breathing. You can stop the internal mental chatter, relax, breathe, and smile. Such a meal can provide many moments of happiness.

A MEAL AT GOOGLE

When I visited Google, I shared a silent meal with some of the people who work there. Afterward, they wrote me and said, "Never before in that cafeteria have I had a meal that wonderful. I was so happy. I felt so peaceful. Nobody said anything in that whole room full of people. Everybody was quiet from the beginning to the end of the meal. In the history of Google, that's the first such meal we've ever had."

ARRANGING A MEAL

You can arrange your schedule so you have enough time to eat. The place and the food should be appropriate. What we eat is very important. Tell me what you eat and I will tell you who you are. Tell me where you eat, and I will tell you who you are.

We are what we consume. If we look deeply into what and how much we consume every day, we'll come to know our own nature very well. We have to eat, drink, and consume, but if we do it unmindfully, we may destroy our body and our consciousness. A meal is an opportunity to show gratitude to those that came before us and those that will come after we are gone.

EATING IS AN ART

Eating well is an art. It doesn't require fancy cooking, but it does require practice and concentration. Your body is not just yours. It is a gift and a responsibility. To keep it healthy, we need to know how to eat.

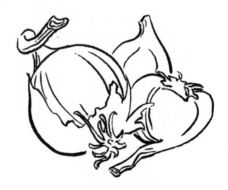

CHOOSING WHAT TO EAT

Our way of eating and producing food can be very violent, to other species, to our own bodies, and to the Earth. Or our way of growing, distributing, and eating food can be part of creating a larger healing. We get to choose.

The planet suffers deeply because of the way many of us eat now. Forests are razed to grow grain to feed livestock, and the way the animals are raised pollutes our water and air. A lot of grain and water is also used to make alcohol. Tens of thousands of children die of starvation and malnutrition every day, even though our Earth has the ability to feed us all.

With each meal, we make choices that help or harm the planet. "What shall I eat today?" is a very deep question. You might want to ask yourself that question every morning. You may find that as you practice mindful eating and begin to look deeply at what you eat and drink, your desire for certain foods may change. Your happiness and that of the Earth are intertwined.

A VEGETARIAN DIET

The Food and Agricultural Organization (FAO) of the United Nations proposed that the meat industry be reduced by at least 50 percent in order to save our planet. The simple act of becoming vegetarian can make a difference in the health of our planet.

If you're not able to entirely stop eating meat, you can still decide to make an effort to cut back. By cutting meat out of your diet even five or ten days a month, you're already helping. Try to reduce your consumption by at least 50 percent. This begins to nourish your compassion. If you know that you're living in a way that makes a future possible for your planet, you'll have joy.

THE PLANET IS US

Our food comes from this beautiful planet. The Earth is inside of us, in each morsel of food, in the air we breathe, in the water that we drink and that flows through us. Enjoy being part of the Earth and eat in such a way that allows you to be aware that each bite is deepening your connection to the planet.

BON APPÉTIT!

Before eating, we wish people will have a good appetite. We say "bon appétit," just as before going to sleep we say "good night." In Vietnamese, they say "please have a sweet, delicious sleep." In Vietnamese, the word "delicious" always goes together with the word "healthy." So delicious food must be healthy food. We eat delicious food in order to have strength and good health. Food that is tasty but destroys our bodies and our minds is not healthy.

When you eat with mindfulness, you consume deliciously. If you don't feel happy, if you don't feel good enough, then you have to inquire of those who've practiced a long time, "Can you help me? How can I taste the moment deliciously?"

ATTENTION TO WHAT WE EAT

Before eating, you may see a condiment dish with red chili peppers. It looks very appealing. But when you look deeper, you know you are sensitive to them, and if you eat them they may affect your digestion. So although they're delicious, they may not be healthy for you. Something can be delicious and not healthy, so we have to be very careful about what we prepare and what we eat. Healthy is good, but healthy and not delicious isn't good either. You have to have both.

BOUND BY A HUNDRED STRINGS

Eating is a practice. The practice must be nourishing for us, for our bodies, and also for our minds. If you eat but you are bound by a hundred strings of worries, anger, irritation, stress, and projects, then these one hundred strings are pulling you in one hundred directions. Your food and your experience of eating will be empty and worthless. So you have to plan properly and have the intention that whenever you eat, you eat in freedom.

MEDITATION AS FOOD

Meditation practice is also a kind of food because it nourishes us. Consider the practice offered by the Buddha to be a kind of food. Any practice must be a kind of food. Walking is like a delicious food. Eating is a delicious food, sitting is a delicious food, and working meditation is also delicious food.

WHAT A BABY EATS

Often when I am giving a talk, a few babies will be in the audience, and some of them will be nursing. The infants don't know what a bell is; they don't understand the word "mindfulness," but they are nourished both by their mother's bodies as well as by the sounds of the bell and the talk. They can feel the collective energy of deep peace as everyone breathes in and out. They are getting many different kinds of nourishing food—the milk from their mothers, the sounds of the bell, and the collective energy of mindfulness all around them.

ORGANIZING A MEAL

We can organize a meal in such a way that it can really be a time of practice. A meal can nourish and heal, be delicious, and also help create a peaceful atmosphere. We have many people who are very good at organizing. They get a lot done during the day. But sometimes they forget to eat! They don't organize their day to include mindful meals. Organizing a meal requires making the time to eat, without distractions and worries. Eat in a way that is relaxing and brings you joy. It doesn't take too much organizing and the results are profound.

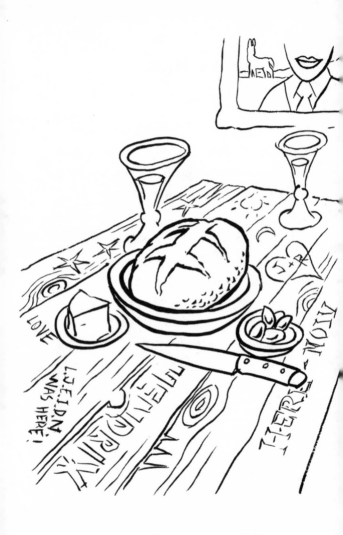

EATING AND SMILING

Sitting at the table and eating with other people is a chance to offer an authentic smile of friendship and understanding. It's very easy, but not many people do it. To me, the most important part of the practice is to look at each person and smile. When family or community members sit together and cannot smile at each other, the situation is a very dangerous one. Upon finishing your meal, take a few moments to notice that you have finished, that your bowl is now empty, and your hunger is satisfied. This is another opportunity to smile and be grateful that you have had this nourishing food to eat, supporting you on the path of love and understanding.

EATING WITH CHILDREN IN SILENCE

Sometimes parents who might want to enjoy a silent meal think that their children will not be able to enjoy or participate in the silence. But children are very capable of eating in silence for five, ten, or even twenty minutes and can enjoy it very much.

CULTIVATING COMPASSION

Having the opportunity to sit with our family
and friends and enjoy wonderful food is
something precious, something not everyone
has. Many people in the world are hungry.
When I hold a bowl of warm, nutritous food, I
know that I'm fortunate, and I feel compassion
for all those who don't have enough to eat
and who are without friends or family. Right
at the dinner table, we can cultivate the
seeds of compassion that will strengthen
our determination to help hungry and lonely
people be nourished.

MINDFUL CONVERSATION AT MEALTIME

I don't recommend that all meals be silent. I think talking to each other is a wonderful way to be in touch. But we have to distinguish between different kinds of talk. Some subjects can separate us, for instance, if we talk about other people's shortcomings. The food that has been prepared carefully will have no value if we let this kind of talk dominate our meal. Instead we can speak about things that nourish our awareness of the food and our being together, cultivating happiness.

Refrain from discussing subjects that can destroy your awareness of the people around you and the food. If someone is thinking about something other than the good food on the table, such as his difficulties in the office or with friends, it means he is losing the present moment and the food. You can help by returning his attention to the meal.

INVITING THE BELL
AT MEALTIME

In our practice centers, we invite the bell
three times before eating, and then we eat
in silence for about twenty minutes. Eating
in silence, we are fully aware of our food's
nourishment for body and mind. In order to
deepen our practice of mindful eating and
support the peaceful atmosphere, we remain
seated during this silent period. At the end of
this time, two sounds of the bell will be invited.
We may then start a mindful conversation with
our friends or begin getting up from the table.

THE PURPOSE OF BREAKFAST

A few years ago, I asked some children, "What is the purpose of eating breakfast?" One boy replied, "To get energy for the day." Another said, "The purpose of eating breakfast is to eat breakfast." I think the second child is more correct. The purpose of eating is to eat.

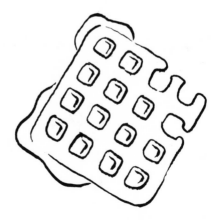

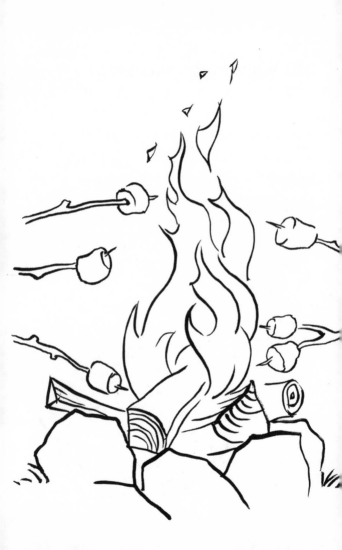

A FULL LIFE

If we feel empty, we don't need to go to the refrigerator to take things out to eat. When you eat like that it's because there is a feeling of emptiness, loneliness, or depression inside. The moments of our daily lives can be filled with joy and meaningful activities. Our community includes our family and friends and our connection to other living beings. They are there to help us get out of these feelings. We are not alone. Sharing a meal together is not just to sustain our bodies and celebrate life's wonders, but also to experience freedom, joy, and the happiness of being in a harmonious community during the whole time of eating.

GETTING SUPPORT

Suppose you have trouble with eating. You eat more than you need to and that has brought you a lot of difficulties and suffering. One way to return to joyful eating is to make a commitment to eat with others who support you. Taking refuge in your community can help a lot. We all need a community to help us in our practice. Even if you live alone and don't have a community to practice with, you are not really alone. Many hands have gone into making the food you're eating. There are the microbes and bacteria and other microscopic living things that are in your food, in you, and all around you. Your ancestors as well as your descendants are with you in every cell of your being.

TRULY SEEING

When we look at the people we're eating with,
we can see them fully in just a few moments.
We don't need two hours to be able to see
another person. If we are really settled within
ourselves, we only need to look for a few
seconds, and that is enough to see our friend.
I think that if a family has five members, only
about five or ten seconds is needed to practice this "looking and seeing."

ENJOYING DISHWASHING

As novices, we had to wash dishes for one hundred monks. There was no running water— no cold water, no hot water, no tap water at all, and no soap. You may wonder how we managed to wash the dishes! We had only ashes, rice husks, and a coconut skin to use as a sponge. Many people in my country still use this. You take a layer of coconut skin and dry it to make into implements for cleaning pots and pans. We had to heat up a big pot of water before we could do any scrubbing. As a novice, I had to go out and gather wood in the pine-covered hills. We gathered dead branches and pine needles into a big heap. You can cook rice or soup with just pine needles.

We were just two novices washing the dishes for one hundred monks. It was a lot of fun washing dishes together, even without hot running water and soap. Some countries have modern homes that are very comfortable. The water, hot and cold, comes right into the kitchen; you have only to turn on the tap.

You can stand there and enjoy washing dishes. But maybe you are lazy. You see a big pile of dishes and you don't want to go over and wash them. But as soon as you roll up your sleeves and stand in front of the basin, it is not difficult anymore.

Whether you are living in a modern country, or you have only a well for water, you can still enjoy washing the dishes.

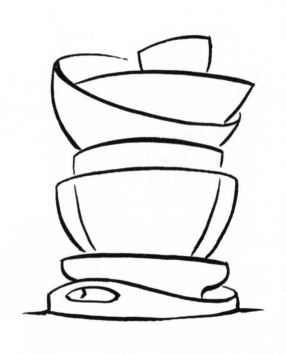

DISHWASHING AS MEDITATION

Suppose the baby Buddha—or the baby Mohammed, the baby Moses, or the baby Jesus—had just been born. You would want to bathe him with clean water. Wash every bowl, every dish as if you are bathing a baby—breathing in, feeling joy; breathing out, smiling.

Every minute can be a holy, sacred minute. Where do you seek the spiritual? You seek the spiritual in every ordinary thing that you do every day. Sweeping the floor, watering the vegetables, and washing the dishes become holy and sacred if mindfulness is there. With mindfulness and concentration, everything becomes spiritual.

DRINKING A CLOUD

Something as simple and ordinary as drinking a cup of tea can bring us great joy and help us feel our connection to the Earth. The way we drink our tea can transform our lives if we truly devote our attention to it.

Sometimes we hurry through our daily tasks, looking forward to the time when we can stop and have a cup of tea. But then when we're finally sitting with the cup in our hands, our mind is still running off into the future and we can't enjoy what we're doing; we lose the pleasure of drinking our tea. We need to keep our awareness alive and value each moment of our daily life. We may think our other tasks are less pleasant than drinking tea. But if we do them with awareness, we may find that they're actually very enjoyable.

Drinking a cup of tea is a pleasure we can give ourselves every day. To enjoy our tea, we have to be fully present and know clearly and deeply that we are drinking tea.

When you lift your cup, you may like to breathe in the aroma. Looking deeply into your tea, you see that you are drinking fragrant plants that are the gift of Mother Earth. You see the labor of the tea pickers; you see the luscious tea fields and plantations in Sri Lanka, China, and Vietnam. You know that you are drinking a cloud; you are drinking the rain. The tea contains the whole universe.

SNACK MEDITATION

A young friend once asked me to teach him about the practice of mindfulness. I offered him a tangerine, but he continued telling me about his many projects—his work for peace, social justice, and so on. While he was eating, he was thinking and talking. He peeled the tangerine and tossed the sections into his mouth and quickly chewed and swallowed.

I said, "Jim, stop! Eat your tangerine." He looked at me and understood. So he stopped talking and began to eat much more slowly and mindfully. He separated each of the remaining sections, smelled their beautiful fragrance, put one section at a time into his mouth, and felt all the juices surrounding his tongue. What is the purpose of eating a tangerine? It is to eat the tangerine. During the time you eat a tangerine, eating that tangerine is the most important thing in your life.

The next time you have a tangerine, please put it in the palm of your hand and look at it in a way that makes the tangerine real. You don't need a lot of time; just two or three seconds is enough. Looking at it, you will see the beautiful tangerine blossom with sunshine and rain, and the tiny tangerine fruit forming. You can see the baby fruit grow and its color change from green to orange. Peeling the tangerine, smelling and tasting it, you can be very happy. Everything we do can be like this. Whether planting lettuce, washing dishes, writing a poem, or adding columns of numbers, we can do it with concentration and awareness.

THE RIGHT AMOUNT

Mindfulness of eating helps us to know what and how much we should eat. We should take only what we can eat. We tend to ignore the rule of moderation. Many of us should take less than what we're used to eating every day. We see that people who consume less are healthier and more joyful, and that those who consume a lot may suffer very deeply. If we chew carefully, if we eat only what is healthy, then we won't bring sickness into our body or our mind.

SNACKING

If we are hungry, a little snack can be very satisfying. But often we develop a habit of eating a snack whenever we feel loneliness or anxiety. A mindful breath is a good way for your body to "snack" on some mindfulness and recognize and embrace strong feelings that may be there. After a mindful breath, you may have less desire to go and fill up with a snack to distract yourself. Your body is nourished by your breath.

EATING OUR FEELINGS

We human beings have many feelings, both positive and negative. Some people tend to eat more when they're joyful, while others tend to eat less. Some people eat when they are sad or upset as a way of eating their feelings, hoping the feelings will go away. Food becomes a craving then, rather than a source of nourishment. If we don't attempt to look deeply to understand our craving, it will grow. When we take the time to take care of our emotions with mindfulness and compassion, then we can just eat. We can enjoy our food without craving and develop a healthy and positive relationship to eating.

NOURISHING OURSELVES WITH MINDFULNESS

We all know that sometimes we open the refrigerator and take out an item that is not good for our health. We are intelligent enough to recognize that. But still we go ahead and eat it to try to cover up the uneasiness within ourselves—we consume to forget our worries and our anxieties and to repress negative energies like fear and anger. Instead of consuming when a feeling of anxiety comes up, invite the energy of mindfulness to manifest. Practice mindful walking and mindful breathing to generate the energy of mindfulness, and invite that energy up to take care of the energy that's making you suffer. If we can practice like this, we'll have enough of the energy of mindfulness to take care of our fear, our anger, and other negative energies.

MINDFUL CONSUMPTION IS FOR EVERYONE

Eating mindfully is a practice that supports ourselves, our families, our society, and the planet, and it is something everyone of any age can do. Leaders of organizations and communities can model responsible and compassionate eating. If you are a mayor, a governor, or a president, you may want to encourage the people you govern to engage in mindful consumption so that you can reduce the violence and suffering in your community.

THE JOY OF EATING

Eating should be very joyful. When I pick up
my food with my chopsticks, with my spoon
or fork, or with my hands, I take time to look
at it for a moment before I put it in my mouth.
If I am really present, I will recognize the food
right away, whether it is an apple, a radish, or a
piece of potato. I smile to it, put it in my mouth,
and chew with complete awareness of what I
am eating. I chew my food in such a way that
life, joy, solidity, and nonfear become possible.
After eating, I feel nourished, not only
physically, but also mentally and spiritually.

CONTEMPLATIONS
FOR EATING

CONTEMPLATING OUR MEAL

Contemplating our food for a few moments before eating can bring us much happiness. We look at the food in a way that the food becomes real. We think about all the people, animals, plants, and minerals and all the conditions that brought the food to our plate. The food reveals our connection with the Earth and all beings. We remember our determination to eat in a way that preserves our health and well-being and the health and well-being of the Earth. The following contemplations and verses can help us practice mindfulness while eating.

PRACTICING WITH THE FIVE CONTEMPLATIONS

The Five Contemplations can be said before a meal to remind us to be fully present for our meal and enjoy it. You can print them out and read them aloud, or you can memorize them. Then they become truly a part of your meal.

But the Five Contemplations aren't just for reading or reciting before the meal. Otherwise, they can become like something we simply check off before we eat, but then we continue to eat as we always have, carried away by our thinking. Throughout the meal, try to live the Five Contemplations. When you practice eating mindfully, you are worthy of the food. The food that has come to your plate is the result of a lot of love and hard work.

THE FIVE CONTEMPLATIONS

1. This food is a gift of the Earth, the sky, numerous living beings, and much hard and loving work.

2. May we eat with mindfulness and gratitude so as to be worthy to receive this food.

3. May we recognize and transform unwholesome mental formations, especially our greed, and learn to eat with moderation.

4. May we keep our compassion alive by eating in such a way that reduces the suffering of living beings, stops contributing to climate change, and heals and preserves our precious planet.

5. We accept this food so that we may nurture our brotherhood and sisterhood, build our community, and nourish our ideal of serving all living beings.

A GIFT OF THE EARTH

THE FIRST CONTEMPLATION: *This food is a gift of the Earth, the sky, numerous living beings, and much hard and loving work.*

The first contemplation makes us aware that our food comes directly from the Earth and sky. It is a gift of the Earth and sky, and also of the people who prepared it. There is a lot of loving work that goes into making a meal. This contemplation puts you in touch with the insight that the one contains the all. When you pick up a carrot, you can see right away that the Earth, the sky, and the whole universe have come together to make that wonderful carrot. Many people have done a lot of loving work and many elements have come together to bring that carrot to your plate. When you put it in your mouth, you can be in touch with the whole universe. A bunch of beets, a head of lettuce, and a loaf of bread all help you to be in touch with the love, hard work, and difficulties that brought the food to you. Even if you are eating by yourself, you are not alone. You are part of a larger community that helped grow the food. In your food you can see the precious presence and work of so many people.

GRATITUDE

THE SECOND CONTEMPLATION: *May we eat with mindfulness and gratitude so as to be worthy to receive this food.*

The second contemplation is about being aware of our food's presence and being thankful for having it. We can't allow ourselves to get lost in the past or the future. We are there for the food and our food is there for us; it is only fair. Eat in mindfulness and you will be worthy of the Earth and the sky.

When we look deeply at the work that goes into growing and preparing our food, gratitude comes naturally. So many hands have been part of bringing our food to the table. Eating mindfully is a way of showing appreciation for all the hard work that has gone into manifesting this meal.

EATING WITH MODERATION

THE THIRD CONTEMPLATION: *May we recognize and transform unwholesome mental formations, especially our greed, and learn to eat with moderation.*

The third contemplation is about becoming aware of our negative tendencies and not allowing them to carry us away. We need to learn how to eat in moderation, to eat the right amount of food. It is very important not to overeat. If you eat slowly and chew very carefully, you will get plenty of nutrition. The right amount of food is the amount that helps us stay healthy.

The Buddha was always reminding his monks to eat with moderation. To eat with moderation means to have a light, healthy body. Many illnesses come to us through our mouths. So we want to look into what we eat, and know what we should eat and what we should not eat. Look with the eye of the Buddha. The quality of the food and the quantity of the food is very important. Every monk and nun traditionally has an alms bowl, which is called "the vessel of appropriate measure." It helps them know how much food to take. When they're offered too much food during the almsround, they give some of it to others. So the bowl helps a lot. We know exactly what quantity of food we want to consume, as well as the quality.

EATING TO REDUCE SUFFERING

THE FOURTH CONTEMPLATION: *May we keep our compassion alive by eating in such a way that reduces the suffering of living beings, stops contributing to climate change, and heals and preserves our precious planet.*

The fourth contemplation is about the quality of our food. We are determined to ingest only food that has no toxins for our body and our consciousness, food that keeps us healthy and nourishes our compassion. When you eat in such a way that you can keep compassion alive in you, that is mindful eating.

Sometimes, even if we're not hungry, we eat to cover up the suffering inside. We can eat in a way that doesn't cover up suffering but acknowledges it and helps it transform.

You may even smile to your own suffering, because suffering has a role to play in helping us transform. Awareness of suffering plays a very important role in helping us to understand suffering and generate the energy of compassion. With mindfulness we're no longer afraid of suffering and pain. We learn how to make good use of the mud of suffering to fabricate lotus flowers.

NURTURING ALL BEINGS

THE FIFTH CONTEMPLATION: *We accept this food so that we may nurture our brotherhood and sisterhood, build our community, and nourish our ideal of serving all living beings.*

The fifth contemplation reminds us to be aware that we receive food in order to realize something. Our lives should have meaning, and that meaning is to help people suffer less and help them to touch the joys of life. When we have compassion in our hearts and we know that we are able to help a person suffer less, life begins to have more meaning. This is an important source of nourishment for us and can bring us a lot of joy. One individual is capable of helping many living beings. This is something we can do wherever we are.

SIX FOOD CONTEMPLATIONS FOR YOUNG PEOPLE

It's wonderful for families to experience the happiness of sitting and eating mindfully together. These Six Contemplations were written particularly to be shared with young people before a meal, but they can be enjoyed by anybody.

1. This food is the gift of the whole universe: the Earth, the sky, the rain, and the sun.

2. We thank the people who have made this food, especially the farmers, the people at the market, and the cooks.

3. We only put on our plate as much food as we can eat.

4. We want to chew the food slowly so that we can enjoy it.

5. This food gives us energy to practice being more loving and understanding.

6. We eat this food in order to be healthy and happy, and to love each other as a family.

SERVING FOOD

In this food
I see clearly
the presence of the entire universe
supporting my existence.

This verse helps us see that our life and the lives of all species are interrelated. Eating is a very deep practice. As you wait to serve yourself or be served, look at the food and smile to it. It contains sunshine, clouds, the sky, the Earth, the farmer, everything.

Look at a peach deeply. Don't put it into your mouth right away. Look at it and smile to it, and if you are mindful you will see the sunshine inside the peach. A cloud is inside. The great Earth is inside. A lot of love and a lot of hard work are inside. Then, when you eat it, please be sure to chew only the peach, and not your projects or your worries. Enjoy eating your peach. The peach is a miracle. You, also, are a miracle. So spend time with your food; every minute of your meal should be happy. Not many people have the time and the opportunity to sit down and enjoy a meal like that. We are very fortunate.

LOOKING AT YOUR PLATE

This plate of food,

so fragrant and appetizing,

also contains much suffering.

This verse has its roots in a Vietnamese folk-song. When we look at our plate, filled with fragrant and appetizing food, we should be aware of the bitter pain of people who suffer from hunger. Every day, thousands of children die from hunger and malnutrition. Looking at our plate, we can see Mother Earth, the farm workers, and the tragedy of the unequal distribution of food.

We who live in North America and Europe are accustomed to eating foods imported from other countries, whether it is coffee from Colombia, chocolate from Ghana, or fragrant rice from Thailand. Many children in these countries, except those from rich families, never see the fine products that are put aside for export in order to bring in money. Some parents are so poor and starving they have to sell their children as servants to families who have enough to eat.

Before a meal, we can join our palms in mindfulness and think about those who do not have enough to eat. Slowly and mindfully, we breathe three times and recite this gatha, or verse. Doing so will help us maintain mindfulness. May we find ways to live more simply in order to have more time and energy to change the system of injustice that exists in the world.

BEGINNING TO EAT

With the first mouthful, I practice

    the love that brings joy.

With the second mouthful, I practice

    the love that relieves suffering.

With the third mouthful, I practice

    the joy of being alive.

With the fourth mouthful, I practice

    equal love for all beings.

During the time we eat the first mouthful, we express our gratitude by promising to bring joy to at least one person. With the second mouthful, we can promise to help relieve the pain of at least one person. With the third mouthful, we are in touch with the wonders of life. With the fourth mouthful, we practice inclusiveness and the love that is characterized by nondiscrimination. After this, we get in touch with the food and its deep nature.

LOOKING AT YOUR
EMPTY BOWL

My bowl, empty now,

will soon be filled with precious food.

Beings all over the Earth are struggling to live.

How fortunate we are to have enough to eat.

When many people on this Earth look at an empty bowl, they know their bowl will continue to be empty for a long time. So the empty bowl is as important to honor as the full bowl. We are grateful to have food to eat and we can find ways to help those who are hungry.

FINISHING YOUR MEAL

My bowl is empty.

My hunger is satisfied.

I vow to live

for the benefit of all beings.

After eating, don't rush on to the next thing. Instead, spend a moment being grateful for the food you have just eaten and all that came together to create this moment. Sometimes we show our gratitude only before we eat, and then after the meal we move on. But we are as grateful for having eaten and for feeling satisfied as we are in the moments of contemplation before we eat. Living peacefully and happily is the best way to show our gratitude and is our greatest gift for the world and the next generation.

HOLDING YOUR CUP OF TEA

This cup of tea in my two hands,

mindfulness is held perfectly.

My mind and body dwell

in the very here and now.

Wherever you are drinking your tea, whether at work or in a café or at home, it is wonderful to allow enough time to appreciate it. If the weather is cold, you can feel the warmth of the cup in your hands. Breathe in and recite the first line; breathe out and recite the second. The next inhalation is for the third line, and the next exhalation is for the fourth line. Breathing mindfully in this way, we recuperate ourselves and the cup of tea reclaims its highest place. If we're not mindful, it's not tea that we're drinking but our own illusions and afflictions. If the tea becomes real, we become real. When we are able to truly meet the tea, at that very moment we are truly alive.

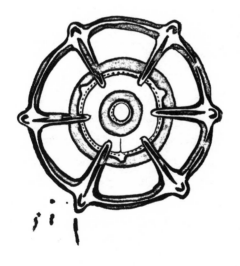

BATHING A BABY

Washing the dishes
is like bathing a baby Buddha.
The profane is the sacred.
Everyday mind is Buddha mind.

When you are cleaning the kitchen or washing the dishes, do it as if you were cleaning an altar or washing a baby. Washing in this way, joy and peace can radiate within and around you. The idea that doing dishes is unpleasant can occur to us only when we are not doing them. Once we're standing in front of the sink with our sleeves rolled up and our hands in warm water, it's really not bad at all. I enjoy taking my time with each dish, being fully aware of the dish, the water, and each movement of my hands. I know that if I hurry in order to go and have dessert or a cup of tea, the time of dishwashing will be unpleasant. That would be a pity, because the dishes themselves and the fact that I am here washing them are both miracles!

If I am incapable of washing dishes joyfully, if I want to finish them quickly so I can go and have dessert and a cup of tea, I will be equally incapable of doing these other things joyfully. With the cup in my hands, I will be thinking about what to do next, and the fragrance and flavor of the tea, together with the pleasure of drinking it, will be lost. I will always be dragged into the future, never able to live in the present moment. The time of dishwashing is as important as any other time.

COMPOSTING OUR FOOD SCRAPS

In the garbage, I see a rose.

In the rose, I see the garbage.

Everything is in transformation.

Even permanence is impermanent.

Whenever we throw food in the compost, it can smell bad. Rotting organic matter smells especially badly. But it can also become rich compost for fertilizing the garden. The fragrant rose and the stinking garbage are two sides of the same existence. Without one, the other cannot be. Everything is in transformation. The rose that wilts after six days will become a part of the compost. After six months the compost is transformed into a rose.

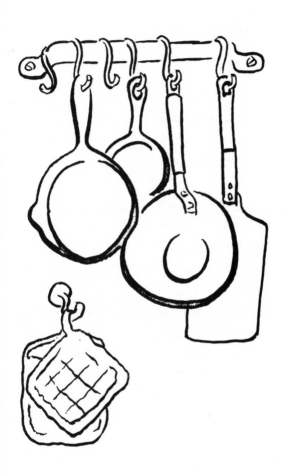

A WAY OUT

I know the Earth is my Mother,

a great living being.

I vow to protect the Earth,

and the Earth protects me.

We practice eating mindfully not just to heal ourselves and our loved ones, but as a way to help the world out of the difficult situation we are in. We become aware of what to consume and what not to consume in order to keep our bodies, our minds, and the Earth healthy, and not to cause suffering for ourselves and for others. Mindful consumption is the way out of our difficulties, not just our personal difficulties, but also the way out of war, poverty, and climate crisis. The Earth requires now that we consume mindfully if we are to survive and thrive as a species.

RELATED TITLES

Awakening Joy
by James Baraz and Shoshana Alexander

Be Free Where You Are by Thich Nhat Hanh

Being Peace by Thich Nhat Hanh

Breathe, You are Alive! by Thich Nhat Hanh

The Cosmos in a Carrot by Carmen Yuen

Deep Relaxation by Sister Chan Khong

Happiness by Thich Nhat Hanh

How to Sit by Thich Nhat Hanh

Making Space by Thich Nhat Hanh

Small Bites by Annabelle Zinser

Moments of Mindfulness by Thich Nhat Hanh

Ten Breaths to Happiness by Glen Schneider

Monastics and laypeople practice the art of mindful living in the tradition of Thich Nhat Hanh at retreat communities worldwide. To reach any of these communities, or for information about individuals and families joining for a practice period, please contact:

Plum Village
13 Martineau
33580 Dieulivol, France
www.plumvillage.org

Magnolia Grove Monastery
123 Towles Rd.
Batesville, MS 38606
www.magnoliagrovemonastery.org

Blue Cliff Monastery
3 Mindfulness Road
Pine Bush, NY 12566
www.bluecliffmonastery.org

Deer Park Monastery
2499 Melru Lane
Escondido, CA 92026
www.deerparkmonastery.org

The Mindfulness Bell, a journal of the art of mindful living in the tradition of Thich Nhat Hanh, is published three times a year by Plum Village.

To subscribe or to see the worldwide directory of Sanghas, visit **www.mindfulnessbell.org**.

PARALLAX
PRESS

Parallax Press is a nonprofit publisher, founded and inspired by Zen Master Thich Nhat Hanh. We publish books on mindfulness in daily life and are committed to making these teachings accessible to everyone and preserving them for future generations. We do this work to alleviate suffering and contribute to a more just and joyful world. For a copy of the catalog, please contact:

Parallax Press
P.O. Box 7355
Berkeley, CA 94707
Tel: (510) 525-0101
www.parallax.org